Esquire's
THINGS A
MAN
SHOULD KNOW ABOUT
Style

Esquire's
THINGS A
MAN
SHOULD KNOW ABOUT
Style

SCOTT OMELIANUK
AND TED ALLEN

RIVERHEAD BOOKS, NEW YORK

Riverhead Books
Published by The Berkley Publishing Group
A division of Penguin Putnam Inc.
375 Hudson Street
New York, New York 10014

Book design by Pauline Neuwirth, Neuwirth & Associates, Inc.
Cover design by Joshua Liberson
Photographs by Brian Velenchenko
Photo editing by Ian Spanier
Styling by Severin and Louise Godwin for Tiffany Whitford, NYC

First edition: October 1999

The Penguin Putnam Inc. World Wide Web site address is
http://www.penguinputnam.com

Library of Congress Cataloging-in-Publication Data
Omelianuk, Scott.
       Esquire's things a man should know about style / Scott Omelianuk
    and Ted Allen: — 1st ed.
          p.   cm.
       ISBN 1-57322-763-3
       1. Men's clothing Miscellanea.   2. Men's clothing Humor.
    3. Grooming for men Miscellanea.   4. Grooming for men Humor.
    I. Allen, Ted.   II. Esquire (New York, N.Y.).   III. Title.
    IV. Title: Things a man should know about style.
    TT617.044   1999
    646'.32—dc21   99-25788
                                                    CIP

Printed in the United States of America

10 9 8 7 6 5 4 3 2 1

introduction

What you don't know could fill a book, wiser men than we have said. And here it is. That book, we mean.

It should come as some small satisfaction to note that it's not all that big of a book. It's also an amusing and pleasurable volume, we hope—something that might yield a quote or two for cocktail parties, or give you reason to chuckle quietly to yourself while riding on an airplane. But a book, nonetheless.

For while there are surely many endeavors about which you are a genuine expert—brilliant, even, at the absolute tip-top of your game, yessir—surely a man as assured as yourself would be the first to admit that there are certain areas about which you do not, as they say, know jack. This is true of all men.

When it comes to, say, 200-thread-count sheets or glass-blowing or piano bars, this ignorance is not only trivial, it's to be admired. But when it comes to dressing well and comporting yourself with style, it *is* a problem, and you know it. It can cost you jobs, women, and friends; it can cause you to be scorned by a maitre d', ignored by an airline-ticket agent, passed up by a taxi driver, and—perhaps worst of all—mocked behind your back by people who actually do know how to match a sock to a shoe to a suit. It can cause you to feel like less of a man than you are, and life is too short to feel like that.

We believe it was Sergio Valente who once said, "How you look tells the world how you feel"—a flimsy, pop-sociological aphorism that could have been spawned only by the seventies, but one that is nevertheless entirely correct. (It should be noted, however, that if you're still wearing Sergio Valente, you're telling the world that you feel like Huggy Bear, the pimp.)

What follows are simple nuggets of truth, lore, exhortation, and caution. These principles do not pretend to comprise the be-all, end-all encyclopedia of matters sartorial. Rather, they are meant as guidelines—basic rules of the road, if you will. Some of which may even be broken, so long as you know what you're doing. Which you don't. Though you will.

—David Granger
Editor in Chief, *Esquire*

Esquire's
THINGS A
MAN
SHOULD KNOW ABOUT
Style

A man in a good suit and tie looks chic;
a man in a good suit without a tie looks more chic.

A man who uses the word "chic"
had better be kidding around.

Jeans must never meet an iron.

There is no foot pain so severe, no dress shoe so fragile, no commute so arduous as to justify the sartorial holocaust that is wearing sneakers with a suit.

In a pinch, paper clips can be used in place of collar stays.

In a pinch, paper clips cannot be used in place of missing eyeglass screws.

That's why you have extra eyeglasses.

Suits are cooler than sports jackets.
And give a short man the illusion of height.

A vested suit can make you look slimmer, or bulkier, depending on the pattern and whether it is tailored correctly.

Never button the bottom button on a vest.

No, no one really knows why.

Well, it's either because (a) the vest's first advocate, Prince Edward VII, left his undone, either inadvertently or because he was fat, or (b) the original full-length vest—also know as a waistcoat—had to be unbuttoned at the bottom to facilitate walking.

If you are one of those men who tends to whistle while prowling the halls at work with your hands jammed into your trouser pockets and jingling the coins therein, stop it.

Unless you want to look lumpy, reduce to an absolute minimum the number and size of the items you carry in your pockets.

Sergio Valente put it best when he said,
"How you look tells the world how you feel."

If you're still wearing Sergio Valente,
you look sort of like Huggy Bear.

With the possible exception of an Ivy League
football game during which people are shout-
ing "boolah boolah" and "twenty-three skidoo,"
it is never, ever acceptable for a person of the
male persuasion to wear a fur coat—not rac-
coon, not fox, not mink.

Certain men's coats, however, can tolerate having
their collars trimmed in a short, subdued fur.

Patchwork rabbit does not qualify as subdued.

The trench, while an excellent raincoat and quite versatile in a pinch, is not a proper winter topcoat.

The Chesterfield coat is.

When you buy a trench: the Burberry.

Shearlings are fine, if a little cowboyish, which brings us to the next subject:

Cowboy boots no.

Cowboy hats: no.

Cowboy shirts: probably not.

Large belt buckles: only if you're a cowboy.

P.S. Don't leave that bolo tie
in your dresser drawer.

You could die.

Someone could find it.

Wearing a suit does not make you "a suit."

Wearing a bad suit or an incorrectly tailored suit or the same damned striped navy suit every day does.

The good suit: horn buttons, hand-stitched lapels, felt under the collar, canvas interlining (stitched, not glued, in place), and a fabric soft enough to wear for twelve hours without making you itch to take your pants off.

There are no bargains.

A custom-made suit is called "bespoke" because it has been ordered, or spoken for, by the customer.

Everyone should own at least one bespoke suit.

Given that bespoke suits take two months to make and can cost five grand and really aren't all that much better than an expensive, high-quality store-bought suit, there's no need to own more than one.

That one suit should be navy, black, or dark gray, and solid.

Because it took two months to make and cost five grand—you need to be able to wear it often and with everything.

Center vent: all-American.

Ventless: Italian, and not for the prodigiously buttocked.

Side vents: rather English. Quite.

Fabrics for easy-traveling suits: nailhead, crepe, tweed.

Fabrics for hot days: cotton, linen, seersucker.

Seersucker: not to be worn by men under fifty
or whose primary residence isn't immediately
adjacent to the county courthouse in a Southern state.

Maximum number of inches that the waist of new trousers can be taken in before the back pockets begin to meet: two.

Gold buttons are not a necessary precondition for a jacket to be worn as a blazer.

In fact, gold buttons are never necessary, Admiral.

When the exchange rate is right, it can be cheaper to buy a plane ticket, fly to Italy, and buy two suits there than to buy them in the States. Plus, you get to go to Italy.

Other things to buy in Italy: Florentine leather goods, Pinader stationery, Acqua di Parma cologne, and, the height of style, a really cool Vespa.

Not all Florentine leather goods are good.

All Vespas, however, are really cool.

Cigars are never stylish
in mixed company.

Smoking, while often fatal, offers many
opportunities for the expression of style,
notably Zippo lighters.

Do not ostentatiously light everyone else's
cigarette all the time. They know how.

Never hold a cigarette between your thumb
and index finger, with the palm up.
Nazis do that.

Style affectations: cigarette case,
pince-nez, hip flask, walking stick.

Should you see a man with a walking stick,
seize it and smack him on the hip flask with it.

Number of neckties you *must* own: one.

Which one? The black knit tie.

A black knit tie coordinates with jeans and a
blazer as well as it does with a French cuffed
shirt and a custom-made suit.

Of course, you're better off with a handful,
all in silk: a couple of dark solids, a handful
of simple diagonal stripes, and one or two natty
small-patterned numbers, such as you'd buy at Hermés.

Woven silk ties generally look
more luxe than printed silk.

The Moscow theory as applied to necktie acquisition:
Anytime you see a necktie you like, buy it. If you decide
to wait and come back later, it will be gone.

The tie tack is to fashion as the
appendix is to anatomy: vestigial.

Hats will make a comeback someday.
It is not that day.

Paisley, too, will be back,
but you could ignore it.

Fanny packs are unacceptable,
if only because they are called "fanny packs."

Baseball caps are for getting the
morning paper. And for baseball.

Thermal headbands keep your ears and forehead warm without mussing your hair or making you look the way you look when you wear earmuffs.

Unless you live in Chicago or Buffalo or International Falls, Minnesota, you must never wear a headband.

Ditto earmuffs.

Button-fly pants are harder to fasten, but easier to unfasten.

To that end: Levi's jeans.

Polar fleece is for exercising and snow-shoveling and—let us not forget—is manufactured from recycled soda bottles.

Polar fleece, while just as warm and at times just as soft as cashmere, will never be as desirable as cashmere.

Better than cashmere: vicuna, which is woven of fibers combed from the chins of llamalike animals living in the Andes, and runs about $3,000 a square yard.

Casual Friday does not excuse the visibility of chest hair.

The best thing about Casual Friday is that
it makes those who decline to observe it
look really, really good.

Jack Kennedy wore polo shirts with
suit jackets.

Jack Kennedy knew *when* to
wear polo shirts with suit jackets.

Good for Casual Friday: Clark's desert boots.

Bad for Casual Friday: moon boots.

Ninety-dollar shoes last half as long as $180 shoes, but $360 shoes will last you your whole life.

Three-hundred and sixty-dollar shoes will not last your whole life if you break their backs by refusing to use a shoehorn.

Three-hundred and sixty-dollar shoes without a shine can look like ninety-dollar shoes.

Women notice shoes.

They also notice nose hair; so should you.

Shoe size matters most at the ball of your foot, not at the toe (where it's O.K. for the shoe to be slightly too big), because the ball is where both your foot and the shoe bend.

Try on both the left and right shoe;
one foot is usually larger than the other.

Never try on shoes in the morning.

Try on shoes at midday.

Snakeskin shoes: no.

Crocodile shoes: doubtful.

> Crocodile shoes in any color
> other than black or brown:
> only if you're Barry White.

White shoes are for tennis.

Exception to the above: white bucks.

Owning a set of golf clubs is not a license
for wearing hideous clothes.

Your eyeglasses should match not only your face,
but your clothing.

A guide: Match your eyeglasses to your belt,
your watchband, and your shoes.

Of course, this gets pricey if you have a lot
of different-colored belts.

But, then: You need no belts in colors other
than black and brown.

Silver, stainless steel, and chrome
watchbands go with everything.

Black or brown leather watchbands don't.

For those in the remedial class—
Black shoes: black band, black belt.
Brown shoes: brown band, brown belt.

It was once considered vulgar for a gentleman to wear a watch, since he might appear overly concerned about the passing of time.

A real Timex is better than a fake Rolex.

The best Timex is the original: the Mercury.

The best leather coats are those made with the fewest, largest pieces of hide.

Trifold wallets bulge more than bifold wallets.

Far from attesting to vast wealth,
a bulging wallet attests to slovenliness.

After all, a really wealthy man lets
his accountant settle his bills.

Plus, a bulging wallet is uncomfortable
and bad for your trousers.

Straw hats are for Kentucky colonels
and gardeners.

Clyde—of Bonnie and—was neither a colonel
nor a gardener and wore a straw hat,
and look what happened to him.

Argyle anything is fraught with peril.

What to do should anyone call you a "dandy":
Open closet. Remove contents. Begin again.

Wearing suits when you don't have to will cause people to think that you have really great suits or that you are really comfortable in suits, or that Sy Syms is your uncle.

Three-button suit: yes. Two-button: yes. One-button: only on a tuxedo.

Speaking of buttons, with two you fasten only the top button; with three it's either the middle or the middle and the top.

Should you find yourself in a four-button suit coat: Unfasten all buttons. Remove. Discard.

A man, unless he is under the age of six,
should not wear overalls.

You know how the outside pockets
of a new suit are stitched shut?
Leave them stitched shut.

This preserves the lean shape of a suit
by prohibiting you from stuffing the
pockets full of stuff.

A good suit treated well shouldn't
be dry-cleaned more than two or three
times a season; a good tuxedo treated well
should never be dry-cleaned.

Cuffs: on suit trousers or any pants you'd wear with a tie, except tuxedo pants.

No cuffs: on jeans and khakis, unless they are pleated, which they should never be.

Khakis that are never pleated: Bills Khakis.

Khakis, which are patterned after military trousers, should never be pleated because military trousers have no pleats and because Humphrey Bogart wore khakis and you can be damned sure his didn't have pleats.

The pleats of trousers that fit properly
will never bulge or gap but will lie flat
against your lap.

Contrary to popular belief, a quirky nonconformity
is not expressed through a Mickey Mouse watch or
a Bugs Bunny tie, because, well, do you know
how many tens of thousands of those things sell each year?

Likewise, wit or humor should never be
expressed through your socks.

Once upon a time labels were worn only on the inside of clothes—those were better times.

Some discreet logos, however, are tolerable on sports clothing: Ralph Lauren's polo player and pony, Lacoste's crocodile, Fred Perry's crest, Brooks Brothers' golden fleece.

Umbrellas: size matters.

While it is acceptable to stow one of those collapsible numbers in your briefcase for emergencies, a well-made, full-sized bumbershoot is a true mark of style.

With a wood handle.

And a sharp, dangerous point.

On the other hand, umbrellas are like fancy gloves: Eventually, you will lose them. Spend accordingly.

Blue jeans: weekends.

Black jeans: weekend nights.

White jeans: with those elf boots
you saved from the eighties.

See also acid-washed jeans—no,
actually, *don't* see acid-washed jeans.

**Unless you're a quarterback,
never wear anything with
your name or number on it.**

A goatee: no.

A soul patch: no.

Elvis sideburns: no.

A ponytail: You're joking, right?
Of course you're joking. Ha, ha.

Slim-fitting clothes are for slim men.

Which means if you're a thirty-six,
you won't look skinnier shoehorning
yourself into a thirty-four. You'll look
skinnier wearing a thirty-six.

Even at a company picnic, the boss
should never subject his employees
to a display of his knees.

The above rule doesn't apply if the boss is a she.

Speaking of shes: The great thing about buying a woman thong underwear is that you get to try it on, too.

That was a joke.

A briefcase is to a man as a purse is to a woman.

If you wear mostly brown shoes, get a brown briefcase; if you wear mostly black shoes, get a black one.

Better: Have one of each.

Backpacks are for students and hikers.

A good leather briefcase cannot
be had for less than $500.

Better a good, nylon canvas
portfolio than a bad leather briefcase.

What's worst about a bad briefcase
is the cheap hardware, which will
scratch and break.

The quality briefcase: full-grain leather,
inside and out; brass hardware; strong locks;
strong, leather strap (when applicable).

Be forewarned: Using an attaché's strap
will cause shiny spots on the shoulders
of your suit coats.

Unless you have a harelip or happen to be
Wilford Brimley, you look exactly half as
attractive with a mustache.

Go to work clean-shaven because you are not
Sonny Crockett and even if you are, *Miami Vice*
was canceled in 1989.

Things to shave: face, head.

Things not to shave: everything else.

If you have a lot of back hair,
you could have it waxed.
Or you could keep your shirt on.

Generally, everybody should keep his shirt on.

Under no circumstances sing the song
"I'm Too Sexy." Not alone. Not in groups.
And particularly not while dressing in
front of a mirror.

**Toupees and comb-overs
betray a level of moral dishonesty
equivalent to the practice of
buttock augmentation.**

If you are going bald,
cut your hair close to the scalp.

Despite the wickedly clever strategies developed by department stores to market such items each holiday season, do not succumb to purchasing a Christmas tie.

Nor a Christmas sweater.

Nor—especially nor—clothing that emits Christmas music.

Likewise there is little reason to wear green on St. Patrick's Day; red, white, and blue on the Fourth; or orange on Halloween.

Socks with sandals and dark socks
with shorts are statements to be avoided.

Sandals? On the beach. In the backyard.

Flat or waxed shoelaces stay tied
far better than round unwaxed ones.

All but the very best dress shoes
now come with round unwaxed laces.
You should replace the laces on those that don't.

Men with pale ankles should
always wear socks.

Men with ankles, period, should
always wear socks.

Men who refuse to wear socks should be prepared
for the consequences of exuding the heady aroma of
a locker room.

Exempt from the above: Italian men or
American men who look Italian enough
to have that certain something that allows
them to wear clothes that no normal man
can wear without provoking laughter.

Besides, your feet will feel cooler
if you wear socks.

Because socks wick away moisture better
than leather, that's why.

The length of one's sideburns is
inversely proportional to one's ability
to rise in the corporate hierarchy.

Unless one works at Graceland.

Shaving is important not only to make you look clean, but so as to avoid sandpapering the face of the person you kiss.

Shaving does not require so much foam that your face resembles a meringue pie.

Shaving is best done in the shower or immediately thereafter.

Shaving is never done with her razor.

> More important: Her shaving is
> never done with *your* razor.

Hide it if you must.

> Special attention: just under your nostrils.
> Just under your lower lip.
> Between your eyebrows.

Acquire a styptic pencil, which won't stick
to your face all the way to work the way
those bits of toilet paper do.

Wear no clothing emblazoned with opinions or exhortations.

If you own any T-shirts with such legends as
"I'm with Stupid" or " 100% Bitch" or
"Nobody Knows Me Like Cosmo,"
please put this book down and back away slowly.

It is far better to arrive at an event overdressed
than underdressed—if you leave early, people
will think you've got somewhere more important to go.

A freshly pressed linen suit doesn't look nearly as good as one that's been worn fourteen times without ever encountering an iron.

The business-shirt wardrobe:
Though some style books would prescribe four white shirts, four blue shirts, etc., it's better to have whatever kind of high-quality shirts you like that are acceptable in your office.

That said, your shirt wardrobe should total at least ten, so that the first five can be in the laundry for a week before you're caught without.

Not all shirt collar styles suit all men.

Long face: spread collar,
button-down collar, tab collar.

Square face: button-down collar,
rounded-point collar.

Round face: button-down, long-point collar.

Oval face: anything but the rounded collar.

Band collar shirts make you look either
stupid or like a priest or like a stupid priest.

The business-shoe wardrobe: You can't go wrong with one pair of plain-toe oxfords in black, one cap-toe or wing tip in black, and one plain-toe or wing tip in brown.

Oxfords is a fancy name for lace-up shoes.

Loafers, which are descended from Indian moccasins and shoes sewn by Norwegian fisherman to wear at sea, are too casual to be worn with business suits.

They are excellent casual shoes, however.

And not bad if you're cruising the North Sea for salmon.

The best loafer: Alden cordovan loafers.

Shoe styles in descending order of dressiness:
formal pumps, plain-toe oxfords, cap-toe oxfords,
wing tip or patterned leather oxfords, loafers, bucks,
espadrilles, Dr. Scholl's sandals, hip waders, oily rags.

Speaking of espadrilles, if you wear them,
you should feel ashamed.

Or French. And ashamed.

No matter what fond memories they evoke of the first time he wore them, there are certain garments from a man's past that he should never seek to wear again: a thin leather tie, rainbow-colored suspenders, those little underwear briefs with cartoon superheroes printed on them.

In fact, wear no funny underwear.

Funny underwear shall be defined as those garments including, but not limited to, neon-colored briefs, boxers printed with lipstick kisses, or any style of skivvies whose fly zone is emblazoned with the phrase "Home of the Whopper."

For those still contemplating the wearing
of funny underwear, think: When you are
removing your pants for the viewing pleasure
of another, do you really want that person to laugh?

Unshined shoes are the
bloodstained hands of style.

Unshined shoes?
O.K., then, how about uncombed hair, unshaven face,
untrimmed nostrils, unbrushed teeth, unwiped . . .
do we need to go on?

Cleanly trimming your fingernails is mandatory.

Having a manicure is acceptable.

Finishing your nails with *any* kind of polish is something Liberace would have done and is, like most matters of style pertaining to the late pianist, unacceptable.

No man should dye his hair.

For all hairstyling products: A little dab will, indeed, do you.

In the unlikely event that a little dab will not do you, get a different hairstyle.

Your hairstyle should require no more time to complete than it does for you to tie your shoes.

When in doubt, go short.

One reason short hair is better: easy styling.

Another reason short hair is better:
less susceptible to "hat hair."

Yet a third reason short hair is better:
You needn't shampoo until it begins to smell.

That was a joke, too.

Problem with short hair:
Frequent haircuts are essential.

Solution: Get frequent haircuts.

A suggestion: Every time you get a haircut,
before you leave, make an appointment for
another haircut, generally four weeks later.

If you favor barbershops over salons—
and you are to be commended for this—
find one that will shave the back of your
neck with hot lather.

Using very hot water to wash your face
causes your pores to open and moisture loss to ensue.

Plus it hurts.

Too much cologne is to style as big hair
is to style as platform shoes are to style
as padded underwear is to style, which
is to say way too much.

What is too much cologne? More than two
squirts of good cologne, or more than zero
squirts of drugstore cologne.

Excluding Old Spice, which will always smell good.

Cologne is applied not to the face (that's
aftershave) but sprayed on the chest,
the back of the neck, the hair, or the
hairy part of your forearms.

The reason for putting cologne in those
places is that hair is the best carrier for scent.

Good mouthwash is overpriced,
but cheap mouthwash is useless.

Breath mints. Not gum.

Tooth-bleaching should be
left to the professionals.

**There should be only one
toothpaste flavor in your
medicine cabinet: mint.**

As essential as your toothbrush,
which is to say, an absolute must:
a nose-hair trimmer.

If this doesn't seem to apply to you now,
give it time—it will.

It can also be used in the ear.

If this doesn't seem to apply to you now,
give it time—it will.

The morning shower is as much about therapy as it is about cleanliness.

Lather. Rinse. Don't repeat. The repeat part is just the shampoo company's attempt to get you to run out of shampoo sooner.

Expensive shampoo smells really good.

Deodorant/antiperspirant, not just deodorant.

Let your deodorant dry a few seconds before putting on your shirt.

There is no substitute for thick,
luxurious, large, high-quality,
100 percent cotton bath towels.

The convention for monogramming towels:
the first letter of her first name, then the first letter
of their last name, then the first letter of his first name,
such that if a woman named Amy were to marry
Steven Spielberg, the monogram would be . . .
Must we spell it out for you?

Leave enough room in your closet so that your suits and shirts hang freely without touching.

Hang suits from shaped wooden hangers.

This prevents a suit's lapels from rolling in on themselves and wrinkling.

If you haven't worn it in the last year, get rid of it.

Do not allow children or pets to enter your closet.

> As you contemplate tattooing yourself
> or piercing body parts, try to remember
> a single T-shirt you bought at a rock concert
> five years ago that you still wear.

George Clooney didn't look as good with
that Caesar haircut as he thought he did.

The gym is no place to be fashion-conscious.

To that end: shorts or sweats, not tights.

Dress for the job you want, not the job you have.

A case where the above rule should be ignored: when the job you have is the chief loan officer at a very conservative bank, and the job you want is to be Mookie, the dancing woodchuck, in a musical adaptation of George Orwell's *Animal Farm*.

If you're not sure whether or not it
looks good on you, it doesn't.

The black cashmere turtleneck
looks good on everyone.

Also: the gray flannel suit.

No level of fitness justifies
wearing a tank top in public.

**No level of fitness—or,
for that matter, drunkenness—
justifies wearing a tank top at home.**

A plain short-sleeved T-shirt
works perfectly well at the gym.

While traveling, two small suitcases are better than one large one.

While two small suitcases are better than one large one, one small suitcase is even better.

Best of all: a Sherpa to carry everything for you.

Stylish luggage is great, but, before you spend a mint, consider what will happen to it after you check it, and know that baggage handlers give special attention to buttery-soft leather only because it suggests valuable and easily fencible goods inside.

Travel essential: mouthwash.
Especially on overnight flights.

At the dry cleaner: Order your shirts on hangers, unless you're traveling, in which case boxed folded shirts are handy.

Pack each suit and dress shirt on
individual hangers and in individual
plastic bags from the dry cleaner;
the slippery plastic reduces wrinkling.

Or, roll clothing rather than folding it,
because each fold is a potential wrinkle.

The best travel suit: "high-twist" wool or wool crepe,
which barely wrinkles and smooths instantly in a
steam-filled bathroom.

Lycra, when used sparingly:
not just for aerobics class anymore.

Besides offering comfort and stretch,
small amounts of Lycra help garments
hold their shape and resist wrinkles.

The correct Lycra proportions: shirts made of
95 percent cotton and 5 percent Lycra.
Suits made of 99 percent wool and 1 percent Lycra.

The two-day business trip: one solid blue suit,
one pair gray wool trousers, one black belt,
one pair black cap-toes, one pair casual shoes,
three versatile ties, two white dress shirts and
one blue or gray, three pair black socks,
three pair underwear, lightweight tan sweater,
lined raincoat.

Roll up two of those ties. Pack them in your
shoes—the ones you're not wearing. Wear the
other tie on the plane.

The weekend getaway: one sports jacket, one
pair dress trousers, one button-down oxford,
light sweater, knit tie, swim trunks, tennis togs,
casual shoes, sneakers.

The plain getaway: jeans, shirt, sneakers, false
mustache and glasses.

If you wear a suit on an airplane and there is a flight delay or cancellation, the ticket agent will help you in a way that she wouldn't if you were in sweats.

The preceding principle also applies to the following situations: at restaurants, in certain nightclubs, taxi-hailing, when being pulled over by a policeman, when shopping for lingerie (unless it's for yourself), and in the office, either for the bossing-about of a subordinate or the receiving of a bossing-about from a superior.

Be not just polite but charming to ticket agents, desk clerks, waiters, bellhops.

On a two-week vacation, be sure that there are laundry facilities at the end of week one, then pack exactly half as much as you otherwise would have.

More travel essentials: Pepto, Aleve, and Excedrin PM; melatonin, which will help you sleep in an unfamiliar time zone.

Travel inessentials: Gas-X, Ex-Lax, and Anusol.

If you need those things, pal, you shouldn't be going anywhere.

Always stay in the kind of hotel that will lend
you an umbrella, should you need one.

Always stay in the kind of hotel that will
press a shirt instantly, anytime, day or night.

Always stay in the kind of hotel that will
bring you a newspaper with your
room-service breakfast.

For the same reason you tip the bartender
for the first round, tip the housekeeper on the first day.

A suede blazer is acceptable, if risky
(no bolo, no boots, no ten-gallon hat).

A leather blazer is not, except when
you've been asked to whack somebody with Joe Pesci.

The Hawaiian shirt: no.

It's acceptable, if you're old, to dress in a way
that makes you appear younger.

It's not acceptable, if you're old, to dress in a way
that makes you appear younger than twelve.

Wearing a sport watch with a suit makes you appear younger.

Wearing sneakers with a suit makes you appear younger than twelve.

Or like a stand-up comedian.

Which brings us to Al Gore.
Even he shouldn't wear a watch
with a built-in calculator.

Button-downs, because of their informal roots, should never be worn with a double-breasted suit.

Button-downs are best worn with a sport coat.

You know how some men wear a shirt with a tie and the shirt's a little too small so their neck sort of curls out over the collar like the end of a German sausage bursting beyond its casing? Don't do that.

Unless you speak with a French accent and sing "Thank Heaven for Little Girls," your wedding day is the only appropriate day to wear a boutonniere.

A black suit with a crisp white straight-collar shirt (not a button-down) and a long solid black tie can be worn to any event where you're requested to wear a tuxedo.

That said, never exercise the option of black-tie optional.

Likewise, black tie is not the sort of dress with which to get "creative."

When in doubt, wear black.

On the other hand, wearing all black, all the time, is the transparent affectation of people who want to be seen as artsy, and who should just quit it.

Though many claim that suits and neckties
inhibit creativity, it's instructive to remember
that Matisse and Einstein did just fine in them.

A suit is not an obligation; it is your protector.

A necktie is not an obligation; it is an opportunity.

Although the preceding two items have
the ring of New Age horseshit, the point is
don't shirk the suit and tie.

Despite their prevalence in country clubs, boat shoes should
not be worn with a navy blazer, Biff.

Skinny men can wear things fat men cannot.

Italian men, even fat Italian men, can
wear things American men cannot.

Tall black men can wear things
tall white men cannot.

A man wears nothing under his kilt.

Which is why a man should never wear a kilt.

Brown suits, while wearable, are touch and go.

Saying that brown is the new black is like saying chocolate is the new vanilla.

People who say that brown is the new black
tend to work in the fashion industry,
which abhors the idea of clothing that
"never goes out of style."

There will never be a new black.

Contrary to popular belief,
not everybody looks better in black.

To wit: Tall, thin men of exceptionally
pale visage look more dead than better.

Green suits are not wearable,
are difficult to match ties to,
and can cause a short man to be
mistaken for a leprechaun.

Short men need the illusion of height, which means:
dark suits, vertical lines, tapered trousers,
two- as opposed to three-button suits,
and the avoidance of the horizontal effect
of pocket flaps and cuffed trousers.

Tall, thin men need the illusion of breadth, which means: plaids, patterns, thick, nonclingy fabrics, looser three-button suits, wider lapels, flapped pockets, cuffed trousers.

Ties with vertical stripes: no.

Fat men: See short men. Plus, seek jackets with only slightly padded shoulders to avoid the appearance of tightness there; avoid bulky tweeds, vivid patterns, and pinstripes, which, like the grid on a globe, only serve to accentuate your rotundity.

Similarly, avoid stripes on tight-fitting shorts, unless it is your intention to delineate the longitude and latitude of your Mercator projection.

No man, not even a figure skater,
should wear sequins.

No man, not even a polo player,
should wear jodhpurs.

No man, not even a scoutmaster,
should wear garters.

Rent no clothing.

Lend no clothing.

Borrow no clothing.

Especially your wife's.

Suspenders, ill-employed, produce wedgies.

When to wear suspenders without a suit or tie:
when you are Robin Williams.

Use of a pocket square generally indicates a sophisticated level of dressing, so long as that pocket square wasn't bought in a boxed set with a matching necktie.

Should you be put off by fluffy-looking, colorful pocket squares, or should you not wish to have another color and pattern to worry about matching with your suit, tie, and shirt, opt for a white linen hanky, and fold it squarely, such that a half inch shows from your breast pocket. Presto.

If you can slip two fingers between your neck and the buttoned collar of a new dress shirt, the shirt will fit comfortably after laundering.

To avoid turning your collar into a garrote:
light starch.

The shirt placket, the belt buckle,
and the trouser fly should all line up.

The shirt placket: the strip of material
sewn to the front of your shirt through
which buttons are fastened.

Speaking of belt buckles,
the point of your tie should never fall below it.

Neckties decorated with golf tees or with the paintings of dead rock musicians coordinate with nothing.

It is never acceptable to loosen your tie, except during the process of its removal.

Loosen your tie by gently working free the knot, rather than pulling the end through the knot, which stretches out your tie.

You are in your car an hour a day;
you are in your clothes from morning to night.
Spend accordingly.

The seat-belt shoulder strap
goes under your necktie.

Good shoes and a good haircut matter more
than a great suit.

You can't smoke a pipe
if you're under forty-five.

You can't wear a fedora if you're under forty-five.

You can't wear a bow tie with anything other
than a tuxedo if you're under forty-five or not
a famous novelist or not a total geek.
Got that, professor?

Still, you need to know how to tie a bow
for formal events, like your wedding.

The best way to master the tying of a bow tie:
Have someone who knows teach you and
then practice incessantly.

This you should do weeks before the day
you actually need to tie it.

On that day, keep a clip-on in reserve,
should your bow-tying skills fail,
which they probably will.

Clip-on regular ties are perfectly acceptable
for gentlemen, but only for those
still in the first grade.

Very few people want to see you in compression shorts,
and those who do might not be your target audience.

Likewise tight,
black leather pants, Mr. Bon Jovi.

Never allow yourself to be seen with
anyone employing a fan, a beret,
a monocle, or spats.

If he's got all four, run and hide.

Silk shirts: no.

Diaphanous shirts: no.

Blousy pirate shirts: unless you're a figure skater.
And even then—actually, *especially* then—no.

Glittery clothing: no.

Knickers: no.

Monograms: Proceed with caution.

>   If you must monogram shirts,
>   do it only on the waist, below
>   the breast pocket, or on the front left tail.

And never forget: Clothing emblazoned with crests
is to be avoided by anyone who isn't a member
of the royal family or Captain Stubing.

Select at your peril eyewear so distinctive and prominent that it becomes your primary feature.

Case in point: Harry Caray, Swifty Lazar, Sally Jessy Raphael, and that dinosaur of a woman in the Old Navy commercials.

Round face: square glasses.
Long face: round glasses.

Sunglasses not only prevent you from squinting (which can eventually result in unwanted wrinkles) but protect you from cataracts.

The reason celebrities wear sunglasses indoors is not because you would otherwise recognize them, which they've long grown accustomed to, but so they don't readily notice *you* recognizing them.

Unless the burden of celebrity is a daily pox upon your life, do not wear sunglasses indoors.

A $250 shirt will look like a $25 shirt
if it is professionally laundered
instead of hand-washed.

Still, ironing correctly is difficult and tedious
and best left to experts.

There is no such thing as a stylish slipper.

Velvet slippers with gold brocade—unless you're over fifty
and incredibly wealthy and feel comfortable in an ascot
and are hosting a jazz-age cotillion in your city home, as
opposed to your various country and island homes: no.

No one should feel comfortable wearing an ascot.

It follows that there is no use for a stickpin.

Ditto for a dickie.

No, a dickie is the neck part of a turtleneck sweater without the sweater part, which one wears under another shirt to give the impression that one is wearing an entire turtleneck sweater.

Yes, a dickie *is* a stupid thing.

You will be happiest if you regard dress shirts as ultimately disposable.

Before you buy one more shirt, have a tailor measure these portions of your person, and commit the numbers to memory: neck, arms, chest.

Other numbers to remember: one-half inch of shirt collar above the jacket collar, one-half inch of shirt cuff, one-and-one-half inches of trouser cuff, two inches more belt than inches on your actual waist.

Despite its presence on the label of every high-quality shirt (and many cheap ones besides), only a few insiders know what "single-needle tailoring" is.

Single-needle tailoring: seams stitched down the outside of a shirt first and then from the inside, using one needle and forming a lock-stitch, which is stronger and prevents the puckering that comes with faster, cheaper, double-needle stitching.

You are now at liberty to forget you've ever heard of "single-needle tailoring."

Cotton/polyester blended shirts don't breathe,
do pucker at seams, and will "pill" after a few launderings.

"Easy-care" is for those who don't.

One definition of the high-quality shirt:
100 percent cotton, or 95 percent cotton
and 5 percent Lycra.

Another definition of the high-quality shirt:
a "split yoke," signified by a vertical seam between
the shoulder blades, which permits custom-shirt makers
to adjust the fit of each shoulder separately.

Yet a third definition of the high-quality shirt:
small, tight stitches, removable collar stays, a button
on the cuff placket, pleats on the sleeve where it
enters the cuff, well-sewn buttons with an extra
one attached to the inside of the shirttail.

One ring, maximum. On a finger.
Not from college.
Not from high school.

Silver or platinum or white gold,
not yellow gold.

Harrison Ford doesn't look as good with that
earring as he thinks he does.

Michael Jordan doesn't look as good with that
earring as he thinks he does.

Captain Hook—all right, on *him*, the earring
looks good.

Karl Lagerfeld doesn't look as good
with that fan, those sunglasses,
that trench coat, that makeup,
that cigarette holder, or that ponytail
as he thinks he does.

The only good tattoo is a very, very small
tattoo placed where no one can see it—
which is to say, why get one?

> A man in a suit without a tie
> can get away with wearing loafers;
> a man in a suit with a tie cannot.

Cheap cashmere is less soft and
more fragile than expensive wool.

Number of goats that sacrifice their
belly hairs for your cashmere sweater: six.

Sweater vests: solids, not argyles,
unless you're off to Andover.

Sweaters, generally: If they're patterned,
which carries grave risks, they must be
patterned on the back as well as the front.

A T-shirt that shows through a dress shirt
is the male equivalent of visible panty lines.

Do not wear button-down collars with
double-breasted suits.

Do not unbutton double-breasted suits
as David Letterman always does.

Think twice about double-breasted suits.

The only thing worse than wearing socks that don't cover one's calves is wearing patterned socks that don't cover one's calves.

If you lose one cuff link,
remove the remaining orphan;
this will make it look like
you've omitted them on purpose
and have insouciant personal style.

Keep a lint roller in your office. And your car.

Also for your office: a small safety pin,
a large safety pin, a sewing kit, a small
bottle of spot remover.

The button-down collar, left unbuttoned: no.

> Unless you're wearing it with a pair of jeans
> or khakis and without a tie, in which case it
> should never be starched or ironed, either.

Always keep a fresh shirt, laundered and pressed,
and a tie in your office.

> Never take a necktie to a dry cleaner,
> who will invariably ruin it.

For formal affairs:
Buy the lightest-weight tuxedo you can find,
because dancing and drinking and scantily clad
women cause such events to become overheated.

Dancing can be hell on your clothes,
your shoes, and your hairstyle.

Dancing is best performed by those who can dance.

Those who can dance know who they are.
Usually.

That said, if she asks, dance you must.

What you find at an outlet store is what other people refused to buy or what some marketing director thinks you will buy because you're the kind of person who shops at an outlet store.

Khakis worn religiously on Friday
are no less a uniform than a
business suit worn the prior four days.

Nonetheless, you can never have too many khakis. Or heavyweight white T-shirts or canvas tennis shoes. For Saturday.

The best canvas tennis shoes:
Jack Purcell sneakers.

Your belt and shoes should match
in color, if not material.

Speaking of color,
there is little use for pink, peach, or teal.

It's not the name on the label or the dollar amount on the credit card receipt but how good you look in it.

One $1,000 suit is a better investment than two $500 suits.

Of course, clothes are not really "investments" because, unlike a Jackson Pollock or a treasury bill, they cannot appreciate. They're clothes.

It's more important to a man's daily life
to have a good tailor than a good doctor.

How to pick a tailor:
Visit the finest men's store in town,
find the best-dressed salesman in the suit department,
ask him where he goes. Then, visit another fine men's store,
and run that tailor's name by the best-dressed salesman there.
Repeat.

How to talk to a good tailor: Present your taste in cuffs,
sleeve length, give at the waist, and roominess in the seat;
and then let him do what he wants.

Tip him generously.

At the tailor's, carry everything you normally
carry: wallet, keys, Mace, etc.

Suit trousers ride on your waist—
about an inch below your navel—
not your hips, like blue jeans do.

Suit trouser bottoms should break on top of
your shoe, so that the crease on the leg rum-
ples just slightly.

If your suit trouser bottoms are too short, you'll
look like Garrison Keillor.

If your suit trouser bottoms are too long:
Charlie Chaplin.

Talented clothing salesmen are an essential part
of selecting the right clothes, but finding such a man . . .
Aye, there's the rub.

> Two elements of style that will outlast
> any man who is smart enough to own them:
> a sterling belt buckle from Tiffany & Co.
> and simple cuff links.

A restaurant meal tastes better
when you're wearing a suit coat.

> When wearing nice clothing in a restaurant,
> order only things that can be eaten neatly
> and with a fork.

Things that particularly do not qualify for the above:
sloppy joes. Soup. Spaghetti. Lobster. King crab claws.

Whether a tie is too fat or too skinny
must be decided by you alone, on a tie-by-tie basis.

When in doubt, ask a woman.

Know that she will often be wrong, too,
and that ultimately, a man is adrift in a
vast sea of complexity and indecision
that he alone must ply.

Never trust a fashion magazine.

Solution for snags on many garments:
Don't cut the errant fiber; rather,
thread it onto a needle and pull it through
the snag so that it hangs on the inside.

Never iron anything that could melt.

The presence or absence of gold stripes
on the lining of neckties that once attested
to a necktie's quality no longer does so.

Testing a necktie's quality:
Dangle it from the narrow blade
and see if it hangs without twisting;
pull from both ends and see if it
returns to original size and shape;
drape it over your arm and make sure
the narrow end is centered against the wide end.

Or you can use this old saw:
If it makes a good knot, it's a good tie.

A safe width for ties: three and a half inches.

A safe length: fifty-six inches.

It is no easier or more comfortable
to wear a sport jacket and trousers
than it is to wear a suit.

If the trousers you'd wear with the sport coat are
more comfortable than the trousers with your suit,
you need a new suit.

Deep in the heart of middle America,
some people are actually wearing those
baggy, printed workout pants again,
and you owe God your deepest thanks
that you have the presence of mind
to not be among them.

Hospital scrubs are an excellent choice
when your destination is your bed
and you are going there alone.

Or if you are Marcus Welby, M.D.

An alternative: Sulka silk pajamas.

Because you never know when Hef might call.

Wait—yeah, you do. Hef will never call,
but have you ever felt Sulka silk pajamas? Mmmm.

The only people who can wear colored shirts
with white collars are obscenely overpaid CEOs
and Donald Trump.

And even they look ridiculous in them, but
who's going to tell them?

Wearing an orange tie will not make you look
like Frank Sinatra.

Wearing an orange pocket square will not
make you look like Frank Sinatra.

Frank Sinatra is dead. O.K.?

If you hang your jacket on a chair and then sit
on the chair and lean back, your jacket will look
as if you hung it on a chair and then sat on the chair
and leaned back.

Drape your scarf on that chair and place
that umbrella on the floor and you're going
to find yourself buying another scarf and
another umbrella real soon.

Fabric weights are the chemistry of style; Wool
pants and a linen shirt or a flannel shirt with a
silk tie are corrosive mixtures.

Jack Nicholson can wear two-tone spectator shoes only because he is Jack Nicholson.

Tom Wolfe can wear ice-cream-colored suits only because he is Tom Wolfe.

And remember: Even Tom Wolfe has his bad days.

Before overindulging in cargo pants, consider the stylistic endurance of painter's pants.

Clothing that reveals your preferences in sports teams and rock bands should be left at home with your parents when you move out.

Clothing that reveals your preferences in institutions of higher education is for jogging and car-washing.

Only professional drivers need driving gloves.

Observing Casual Friday tells the world
that you're only confident enough to wear
what you're told you can wear.

On the other hand, we suppose that we are
telling you what to wear, aren't we?

Casual Friday was invented to
embarrass well-dressed men.

Really well-dressed men are not affected by this.

Men named Chick tend to wear
shoes with stacked heels.

Shoes with stacked heels,
like the name Chick, are inappropriate for men.

Woven shoes are for men with small feet.

Think twice about woven shoes.

Plain-toe shoes make big feet look bigger
than do cap-toe shoes or wing tips.

Cowboy boots make big feet look bigger still.
Plus they have stacked heels. Plus they're cowboy boots,
for God's sake. And didn't we already tell you about
cowboy boots?

Of course, plain-toe shoes aren't as bad as
those big red floppy clown shoes, which
make your feet look *really* big. But in a good way.

Don't attempt the tango in clown shoes,
unless you are a trained professional.

If you are a tango professional, man,
what on earth do you need our help for?

If you are a tango professional,
please donate this book to someone
less well-endowed in the style department.